FOOD ADDITIVES

THE EFFECTS OF PROCESSED MEALS AND

ITS ADDITIVES

DR. MAXINE SKINNER

Table of Contents

CHAPTER ONE

Food components

Meals additives are chemicals introduced to meals to maintain them sparkling or to enhance their color, flavour or texture. They will include meals colourings (inclusive of tartrazine or cochineal), flavour enhancers (together with MSG) or pretty a number of preservatives.

Most food components are indexed at the product label, together with specific substances, in a descending order through weight (flavours are an exception and do now not want to be diagnosed). Occasionally, the additive is spelt out in full. At distinctive times, it is represented through a code range: for example, cochineal can be listed as Colouring (100 and twenty); sodium sulphite can be shown as Preservative (221).

Meals additives are components which are introduced to food to perform precise talents.

Manufacturers need to provide facts approximately any components used within the foods they produce. You could find out this information in the listing of substances on the packaging. It's going to let you recognize what every additive does, determined with the aid of manner of its call or E range.

Results of food components

Some human beings are sensitive to specific food additives and may have reactions like hives or diarrhoea. This doesn't advocate that every one meals containing components want to be automatically dealt with with suspicion. All ingredients are made up of chemicals and food components are not typically 'plenty less cozy' than manifestly occuring chemical substances.

Many of the food additives utilized by the meals enterprise also arise genuinely interior ingredients that people devour each day. For instance, MSG is discovered certainly in parmesan cheese, sardines and tomato in drastically greater quantities than the MSG gift as a meals additive. Humans with food allergies and intolerances are also regularly sensitive to chemical compounds decided glaringly in sure meals, which encompass nuts or shellfish.

Many humans view food additives as a first-rate meals hazard. However, in terms of health threat, meals additives may come in at the stop of the road, after food-borne microorganisms (like salmonella), inappropriate hygiene and consuming conduct, environmental contaminants and evidently occurring pollutants.

Styles of meals components

The wonderful styles of food additive and their makes use of encompass:

Anti-caking entrepreneurs – stop additives

from turning into lumpy.

Antioxidants – save you food from oxidising, or going rancid.

Artificial sweeteners – boom the surprise.

Emulsifiers – save you fat from clotting together.

Meals acids – hold the proper acid level.

Colors – beautify or add colour.

Humectants – maintain ingredients moist.

Flavours – upload flavour.

Flavour enhancers – growth the electricity of a flavour.

Foaming agents – maintain uniform aeration of gases in food.

Mineral salts – decorate texture and flavour.

Preservatives – stop microbes from multiplying and spoiling the meals.

Thickeners and vegetable gums – decorate texture and consistency.

Stabilisers and toning sellers – hold even food dispersion.

Flour remedy – improves baking fantastic.

Glazing agent – improves appearance and can protect food.

Gelling sellers – regulate the feel of components through gel formation.

Propellants – help propel food from a container.

Raising stores – boom the amount of food

through using gases.

Bulking dealers – boom the extent of meals with out fundamental modifications to its available electricity.

Meals additives and processed meals

There may be a commonplace misconception that processed meals mechanically contain food additives. Food like prolonged-lifestyles milk, canned food and frozen meals are all processed, but none of them want extra chemicals.

If you are unsure whether or not or no longer a product includes an additive, test the label. However, some indexed elements can also include food additives without mentioning them at the label. For example, 'margarine' might be a indexed element and margarine incorporates meals components.

A few food additives can cause reactions

For the general public, additives are not a problem inside the short time period. However, 50 of the 4 hundred currently approved components in Australia were associated with negative reactions in some people. A few meals components are much more likely than others to purpose reactions in sensitive human beings.

It is regularly the components which are used to present a food a marketable exceptional, consisting of colour, that most normally cause allergic reactions. A number of those allergic reactions encompass:

Digestive problems – diarrhoea and colicky pains

Apprehensive problems – hyperactivity, insomnia and irritability

Respiration problems – allergies, rhinitis and sinusitis

Pores and skin problems – hives, itching, rashes and swelling.

It's far important to understand that the various signs and symptoms professional because of meals sensitivities can be because of other problems. Scientific diagnosis is essential. If you try to diagnose yourself, you could limit your food plan unnecessarily and overlook an infection.

A few common meals components which can cause issues

Some meals components that would purpose problems for some humans include:

Flavour enhancers – monosodium glutamate (MSG) 621

Meals colourings – tartrazine 102; yellow 2G107; sunset yellow FCF110; cochineal one hundred twenty

Preservatives – benzoates 210, 211, 212, 213; nitrates 249, 250, 251, 252; sulphites 220, 221, 222, 223, 224, 225 and 228

Artificial sweetener – aspartame 951.

Diagnosing meals additive sensitivity

If you assume you can have a meals additive sensitivity, it's critical to are in search of for expert help on account that each one the signs you'll be experiencing also can be as a result of different disorders.

It may help to hold a food diary and notice carefully any terrible reactions. In the case of a sensitivity being identified, the same old exercising is to get rid of all suspect ingredients from the food plan and then reintroduce them one at a time to look which additive (or additives) reasons the response. This ought to best be carried out under clinical supervision, considering some of the reactions – inclusive of allergies – may be excessive.

CHAPTER TWO

How we make sure meals components are at ease

Additives need to be assessed for safety before they may be used in food. We additionally ensure that:

The technological know-how on additives is exactly reviewed

The law is precisely enforced

Movement is taken wherein troubles are determined

We look at any information that casts reasonable doubt on the safety of an additive.

Food colorings and hyperactivity

We funded studies into viable hyperlinks among meals hues and hyperactivity in kids. It determined that eating certain synthetic food colors should motive multiplied hyperactivity in some kids.

Those artificial colorings are:

Sunset yellow FCF (E110)

Quinoline yellow (E104)

Carmoisine (E122)

Allura purple (E129)

Tartrazine (E102)

Ponceau 4R (E124)

Food and drink containing any of these six

hues should bring a warning on the packaging. This will say 'also can have an negative impact on activity and attention in youngsters'.

We encourage manufacturers to artwork within the path of finding options to the ones sunglasses. A few manufacturers and stores have already taken motion to get rid of them.

It's crucial to keep in mind that hyperactivity additionally can be as a result of specific matters. So being cautious about what a infant eats may moreover help manipulate hyperactive behaviour but it cannot prevent it.

E numbers

A meals additive is simplest permitted if; it's been tested and proved to be cozy for its intended use; there may be a justifiable technological want to use it; and its use does no longer deceive the consumer.

All of the components we eat include chemicals in a single shape or each other. Many meals additives are chemical substances which exist in nature along with antioxidants ascorbic acid (diet C) or citric acid, discovered in citrus end result.

Due to technological advancements, many other additives are now guy-made to carry out sure technological skills. Whether or not or no longer the chemical compounds utilized in components exist in nature, they're problem to the identical safety evaluations.

A few consumers think about meals additives (E numbers) as a contemporary invention used to make reasonably-priced meals. In fact, meals components have an extended records of intake and are utilized in lots of traditional food. As an instance, wines such as Champagne consist of sulphites, and 1st Baron Verulam consists of the preservatives nitrates and nitrites to prevent the growth of botulism.

Sweeteners

As with every special food components, sweeteners need to undergo a protection assessment earlier than they'll be permitted for use in meals.

Great individuals who are recognized at start with phenylketonuria need to keep away from ingredients containing certain sweeteners, i.E. Aspartame and aspartame-acesulfame salt. This is because they can't devour ingredients containing phenylalanine which includes components inclusive of meat, dairy and nuts.

Because of stated issues about sensitivity to aspartame (e.G. Complications, dizziness and stomach upsets) the meals necessities agency commissioned studies to analyze this similarly. Those who self-reported sensitivity to aspartame had been either given a cereal bar without or with aspartame; but have been no longer instructed which bar they'd fed on. The effects confirmed that there has been no difference in cited symptoms after eating the aspartame containing bar in assessment to the regular bar.

Glycerol

Slush ice drinks can incorporate the detail glycerol as an alternative for sugar, at a diploma required to create the 'slush' impact. At this diploma, we advocate that children aged four years and under have to not devour those drinks.

This is because of their capability to purpose aspect-outcomes which include headaches and illness, specially when consumed in more.

Caffeine in 'power drinks' and other substances

Strength liquids are normally beverages with excessive-stage of caffeine that producers say come up with greater 'energy' than regular gentle beverages like cola. They're unique to 'sports sports drinks' which you may use to update electrolytes out of place at some stage in exercising.

Electricity drinks can comprise excessive levels of caffeine, normally about 80 milligrams (mg) of caffeine in a small 250ml can – that's what you would discover in two or three cans of cola or a mug of immediately coffee. There are also big 500ml cans to be had which comprise approximately 160mg of caffeine. Some of the smaller 'energy shot' merchandise can consist of everywhere from 80mg to as a bargain as 160mg of caffeine in a 60ml bottle.

THE END

www.ingramcontent.com/pod-product-compliance
Lightning Source LLC
Chambersburg PA
CBHW061931270726
48660CB00003BA/1131